LIVE HEALTHY WITH CROHN'S DISEASE

*13 Aspects to Managing your Disease
to live a symptom-free life*

Rebecca Renck

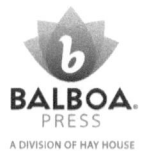

BALBOA
PRESS
A DIVISION OF HAY HOUSE

Balboa Press books may be ordered through booksellers or by contacting:

Balboa Press
A Division of Hay House
1663 Liberty Drive
Bloomington, IN 47403
www.balboapress.com
1 (877) 407-4847

Print information available on the last page.

ISBN: 978-1-5043-5695-4 (sc)
ISBN: 978-1-5043-5696-1 (e)

Library of Congress Control Number: 2016907629

Balboa Press rev. date: 05/23/2016

Introduction

A Little about Me

I am a fifty-five-year-old mother of four who was diagnosed with Crohn's disease and inflammatory bowel disease (IBD) twenty-five years ago at age thirty.

I have endured all the typical physical symptoms of this disease, including debilitating pain (the kind where you can't take a breath), diarrhea, constipation, cramping, bloating, gas, fatigue, anemia, malnutrition, medication side effects, and weight loss. I have suffered the emotional traumas that come with ill health—embarrassment, insecurity, fear, frustration, and the unknown.

When I was diagnosed, I had four stomach ulcers, a constricted duodenum, and six acute inflamed areas of colon. I had lost twenty pounds and was so malnourished that walking up the stairs had me sitting and resting at the top. I was placed in the hospital for a week and treated with steroids, which was the only acute medication option at the time. The most acute symptoms subsided, and I was ecstatic in the drug induced-high, believing all my problems were solved and my good health would soon return. I quickly realized the fallacy in the belief that feeling good was healing. My real issues with this disease had just begun.

Not being a fan of the medication regimen or surgery prognosis I had been given by the doctors, I started to look outside the box at this disease that was causing me so much distress. Even with the active, acute symptoms I was experiencing, I made the decision very early in my diagnosis that, if I could, I wanted to manage this disease without surgeries or strong medications. In fact, I refused to believe that those treatments were even an option for me. I had no idea how I was going to accomplish this or what it would look like over my lifetime. I had the intuition that part of the problem was emotional and part was physical (I had given birth to four children in six years and was eating a very standard American diet) but was rather lost as to what I needed to do every day to help myself.

This diagnosis was quite a shock to me and the healthy family I came from. My family loved me but had no idea what I was going through or how to help me—other than to tell me, "Do what the doctors say." I did not want to be sick, but did not want surgeries or lifelong medications to be my future either. I wanted a normal, healthy body. I wanted to live a normal, healthy life. But as is so often the case, the rosy picture of my future needed to be redefined, and I believed a big part of the that definition was to find out how to take care of myself. The path I decided to take was neither the conventional one nor the easiest one, but the end result has been well worth the struggle, and well worth the journey. I found a peace in taking care of myself that I did not know was missing. I found confidence in my intuition. I found a strength in my body that served me well, and I found my health. I was a believer in conventional medicine, but I am now a bigger believer in the ability of each of us to heal our bodies through our thoughts and actions.

I was very strong in my belief, but it was not easy in the earlier years. At times I suffered the ridicule of my family. I had to make some very unpopular decisions, and I have spent many hours researching. I have supported my determination with faith and self-development growth. I sought out the best advice on conventional medicine, nutrition, spirituality, stress relief, and taking care of myself. It has worked. I have lived through actively raising children, being a volunteer in numerous organizations, owning a family business, enjoying being an outdoor camp director, holding two jobs with kids in three different schools, being divorced, and losing family.

In short, I never let the disease stop me. Looking back, I didn't suffer more than needed. The symptoms I had increasingly became mild enough that never more than a six- to eight-week dose of steroid treatment was needed to get the inflammation reduced and the Crohn's in remission. Eventually, I could pinpoint the lifestyle choice or event that caused flare-ups, and I was able to calm my gut down by being aware of it and by making needed changes without the medicine. Over the years, it was gratifying to see that my lifestyle was working and that I had very little active disease. Since I have not neglected going to the doctor for the routine check-ups and tests, I have found that I am actually healthier as the years go by.

I am now here to help you. In 1990, Crohn's was not a well-known disease. I am disheartened that in the past five to ten years, the numbers of those who suffer with Crohn's has grown exponentially. I am heartbroken to think of all the Crohn's sufferers out there who are giving in to surgeries and strong medications, thinking those treatments are their only option. I am living proof that the disease management can be different. It is my goal to reach out to you so you can have the knowledge to make an informed choice about your health. Not to discredit it altogether, but very often conventional medicine makes us believe we have no choice but to follow their standard of care. By definition, Crohn's disease does not have a cure, so the best doctors can do is to help us manage the symptoms with the tools at their disposal. I am here to offer you some additional tools; tools that offer you control of your own health without your feeling dependent upon or the victim of conventional medicine; tools that will bring you success. It has worked for me, and I believe it can work for you, too.

The Reality: You Can Heal Where the Doctors Can't

You have been diagnosed with something called Crohn's disease, inflammatory bowel disease, ulcerative colitis, or any of the other names this malady has been given. You have looked at all the scary literature and heard the dire medical advice and prognosis (no cure, live with it).

What do you do now? Maybe you have acute symptoms and are enduring the debilitating effects of pain, fatigue, diarrhea, medications, and surgery. Or maybe you are in a remission. Your symptoms have subsided, but you are worried about when the next attack will be. Wherever you are in your journey, it is my hope that you can believe it can be better. Life with Crohn's is not easy. You may find that the journey recommended in this book is not an easy one either, but it *will* be worth it, and it *can* give you the normal, healthy life you so want and deserve. You are the one in control, and your decision will give you the strength to make the everyday choices that will eventually lead to a symptom-free and disease-free everyday life.

It is time to take responsibility for your own health and well-being. Just as one could not expect a doctor or a medication to cure heart disease, you cannot expect a doctor or medications to cure your Crohn's disease. Doctors and medications can do nothing to help what I believe are the main causes of the disease: your lifestyle choices, beliefs, and emotional reactions. Diseases come from dis-ease in your body, and dis-ease is the result of your lifestyle. Whether you are aware of all the causes right now or not, you do need to take responsibility, not only for the dis-ease but also for the healing. As you take responsibility for where you are today and then decide you can heal your body, you will learn what you need to learn and do what you need to do. Eventually you will find comfort in the success you will achieve, and that makes all the difference.

Conventional medical treatments and medications work only for a time. Surgery works only for a time. Doctors can only do so much. What I want to share with you can work *for a lifetime*. You can heal where the doctors can't.

When you were diagnosed with Crohn's disease, you may have been given any number of causes of the disease—or maybe none at all. Today, you may hear something like this: "while the exact cause of Crohn's remains unknown, researchers now believe that a combination of genetics, environmental factors, and an abnormal immune response may result in damaging inflammation of the digestive tract." There is no mention of emotions or stress being an issue. What environmental factors are in play? What is an abnormal immune response? Can I change this? This typical explanation only raises more questions.

Was I born with this? Is it stress? Is it diet? Is it living in the city? Is it living in the South or the West? Is it my relationship? What am I doing wrong? How can I fix this? Conventional medicine is giving us few answers.

It is my belief that the causes of Crohn's disease are both physical and emotional stresses that have overrun our bodies. The body's reaction is inflammation. The physical stresses affect the whole body, reducing the effectiveness of the immune system and impairing the physical body from functioning correctly. Emotional stresses have landed in your digestive tract and also caused your physical body to malfunction. For healing to be achieved, the causes of both the physical and the emotional stresses must be identified and then eliminated one by one.

Crohn's affects one of our most basic bodily functions—taking in food and eliminating waste. While it may be chronic and incurable, it is described as *manageable*, which by definition tells me that I can do something about this. I have found that to be true—but you do need to pay close attention to your gut and to what makes it hurt. You need to look at your life and emotional reactions and see what is causing the dis-ease. No matter where you are in the diagnosis, you are not past the point of no return, and any change will make a difference starting today. The work is in finding what makes a positive change to your lifestyle that will, in turn, make a difference in your health. This is what you will find in this book. I want to explore the fact that there are causes for this disease. Then I want to share some tools that I have found are successful—tools that will help you adjust your beliefs and lifestyle, reduce the symptoms, and heal your body.

The reality is that this disease is a good thing in your life, a wakeup call, a blessing. You could argue that having to run to the nearest bathroom, experiencing pain after eating every bite, or staying home to sleep after barely making it through your workday instead of being out with friends are not good things. You would be correct on all accounts. *But* I am here to offer a different perspective—a perspective that will offer you a chance to see why you are suffering from this disease, how you can take back control of your gut, and why it is a blessing in disguise.

The reality is that the life you have led, the emotions you have felt, and the beliefs that you have lived by have, in fact, gotten you to this place of dis-ease.

You will need to do some deep thinking, some letting go. You will need to make some hard decisions and in the end choose to be healthy. What I am offering here is a roadmap with the tools needed to create a joyful, symptom-free life. The work is yours, and the success will be yours too.

A Common Denominator

We need to love ourselves, our friends and family, our food, our jobs, our ambitions, and the world around us.

You will not hear from your doctor that autoimmune diseases have both physical and emotional causes. We will investigate both of these causes in the tools presented here. My main focus and what you need to be aware of in all the descriptions, practices, and steps presented is that love is the common denominator in this healing process.

It is generally accepted now that our thoughts and emotions are energy. Love is the highest and lightest energy of all. It is where our emotions and physical lifestyles need to start from. We need to love ourselves, our friends and family, our food, our jobs, our lifestyles, and the world around us. Anything less is going to cause dis-ease in the physical body. Luckily for you, it shows up in your digestive tract.

Some of the tools and ideas offered here you may be able to implement right away; some take years to implement. The definition of a lifestyle is that it is long-term and sustainable, and you will need to make any changes in your life with this in mind. There are no quick fixes as lasting change takes time.

If you see yourself needing a different attitude, different eating habits, or a cleaner environment, know that taking the first step will be the hardest. It could also be this first step is the lasting step that makes all the difference, the quick path to get on the main road. It is all a part of the process and no different than anything else in life.

It may be exhausting to think about starting, taking action on, or even trying anything new that promises to make a difference—especially when you feel lousy and as I used to describe it "are barely hanging on by your fingertips." But I also know that you will reach a breaking point. If you are currently at that breaking point, ready to take control, have had enough, and are ready to love yourself enough to be serious about not being a victim to this disease anymore and have just an ounce more energy than yesterday, then *now* is the time to start this process. Make the decision today to do better by yourself. That last ounce of energy will be well spent.

As we go through the following steps that will become the tools to allow you to manage your disease and heal your body, realize I cannot give you absolutes. Since Crohn's disease and IBD (and for that matter *all* diseases) are such personal matters and present themselves differently in each individual, I cannot say, "Do this three times per day, go here weekly, or eat this and it will all be better." What I am giving you is awareness and guidelines to make lifestyle changes that will help you realign your beliefs and work from that energetic, loving place each day.

It is prudent to remember also that the steps are not in a specific "do this," one, two, three order but that they are all part of our roadmap to success. I would recommend that you read through all the steps first, find what is resonating with you, and begin that process. Work your way through the steps as you feel called, but do them all. I have placed the steps to do with our physical bodies first only because these are sometimes much easier to get a handle on. If you find yourself skipping over a step, it is possibly because there is a fear of tackling that process. A word of advice is to pay particular attention to it and put some extra effort toward that step.

It is true that the life you have led, the emotions you have felt, and the beliefs that you have lived by have in fact gotten you to this place of disease. It was not an overnight issue that got you here, and it will not be an overnight fix. I am just now realizing that over the last twenty-five years, I have made thousands of choices with regard to my own good health. Over time it becomes second nature to put your health first and make decisions based from love. This is the foundation of reducing the symptoms, healing your body, and taking control of your disease.

THE PHYSICAL
STRESSES

1

The disease and conventional medicine

The goal is to rely less and less on the conventional medical treatment and more and more on yourself and your lifestyle to manage your disease.

Crohn's disease is classified as both an autoimmune disease and an inflammatory disease. This means that there is an abnormal immune response by one's body that attacks substances and tissues that are normal to the body. Stated another way, your body thinks of itself as a threat. The inflammation is the response of the affected tissue. Which tissues are affected create the symptoms that are caused and the designation of which disease you are suffering from. These sets of diseases (and there are over 150) are also classified as having no cure but can be managed—managed, as in the symptoms and destruction of the tissues involved can be slowed, but the underlying condition cannot be cured.

So the doctor comes from the point of view that there is no known reason or cause of autoimmune diseases and that there is nothing conventional medicine can provide that will sustainably heal your body or cure it from this disease. No doubt you have seen a doctor, been run through some tests, and been diagnosed with this disease due to the symptoms or destruction that it has caused in the digestive tract, and then you were prescribed some medications. Conventional medicine treats symptoms. Medications and surgeries let the body recover to a certain extent, but they do so by basically stopping your body from doing what the digestive tract was meant to do. They cannot cure the disease. Despite some measurable improvement, the reality is that there has been no sustainable healing. The causes have not been addressed.

I want you to see the physical symptoms you are experiencing as a sign letting you know there is an unhealthy issue in your life that is affecting your body. This is where sustainable healing can begin. This issue can be any number of profound things. It could be physical issues such as allergens, bacteria, toxins, chronic dehydration, malnourishment, or sleep deprivation or emotional issues such as stresses, anxiety, frustration, impatience, feeling overwhelmed, disappointment, worry, anger hatred, jealousy, insecurity, guilt, unworthiness, fear, grief, depression, or powerlessness.

With this said, I encourage you to take the medications that have been prescribed until you feel you do not need to. Slowing the tissue destruction process by reducing the inflammation needs to be your first step, and medications are good for this. This will allow your body to recover some and help your mind and emotions to be in a better place. The alternatives I present here are to be first used in conjunction with and in addition to your conventional medical treatments. You need to start today with where you *are* today.

The goal is to rely less and less on the conventional medical treatment and more and more on yourself and your lifestyle to manage your disease. I want to impress on you that as a society we have become overly dependent on conventional medicine to fix our every ailment. The reality is that you can do what the doctors can't. You can heal your body and create a sustainable, healthy, symptom-free lifestyle—for the rest of your life. You can keep your body healthy by seeing what is making it unhealthy and adjusting accordingly.

Putting It into Practice

Step 1—Medications with a Grain of Salt

One of the doctor's responsibilities in conventional medicine is to listen to the symptoms you describe and then match those to a medication shown to stop or mask those particular symptoms. Many times, as it is well known, a medication may do its job in one area of the body but cause many side effects in others.

In your new healing lifestyle, *your* responsibility is to do the following:

1. Do your due diligence on the medications and the disease itself—know the side effects, treatment plans, surgeries, and presumed outcomes, dosages, administrations, and prognosis.
2. Spend time really thinking about your beliefs, your desires, and your life to know how it will affect you both physically and emotionally if any of the treatments work for a time and then don't. What are the side effects, and what will they do to you long term? What is the cost monetarily and to your psyche? This personal research is meant to create confidence so you can be willing to say, "*No*—that is not what is right for me, my body or my lifestyle," and make an informed decision when the time comes.

I personally could not have submitted to a drug administration or a surgery that I was fearful of, that took time each day to remind me of how ill and diseased my body was, or that had long-term side effects that I knew would cause trouble—more dis-ease in years to come. Over the years I refused several medical treatments that were the "new thing" and promised superior results but I felt were not right for me due to side effects or how they were administered. With my constant resolve to find the *issue* to the symptom I was experiencing, I found I could heal without the strong medications.

This is a choice you will need to make for your own situation, but make it informed and with determination and confidence that you know what you are getting into. Do not settle for additional symptoms to satisfy what is only conventional treatment if you do not feel comfortable with that. Do not blindly put your healing in another's hands, only to be disappointed and become distrustful if it does not have the desired effect.

2

Diet and Nutrition

You need to be aware of how nutritious your diet is or isn't and adjust accordingly.

Your doctor may or may not endorse the fact that diet plays a major role in Crohn's management. Many doctors still hide from any nutritional and diet advice, but in our Crohn's symptom world, we know that different foods seem to be good for us and others not so much. What I want you to become aware of goes much deeper than whether a certain food is causing immediate symptoms or not. It is the *nutrition*, or lack of it, and the *poisons* in foods that we need to be aware of for long-term, sustainable healing in our bodies.

There are several important concepts I want to acknowledge in creating our healing and sustainable lifestyle where food is concerned:

- **Foods themselves are not the root cause of the disease**. Your body is reacting to chemical pesticides and fertilizers, GMOs, and toxicity as dangers. These allergens and toxins in foods send the immune system into overdrive, which is by definition an autoimmune disease. Over time these processed, toxin-ridden foods will cause every person some kind of disease in his or her body. At the very least you need to stop bombarding your body with things it is constantly having to fight against.

- **Strengthening the immune system** is crucial. Anti-inflammatory foods and natural supplements with immune-boosting properties need to be a staple in your diet.
- **The human body is constantly regenerating new cells.** This is what sustains our lives and either our ill or good health. To heal and sustain good health, it is crucial to supply new cell development with the most nutritious, toxin-free substances we can. Good, clean foods that supply the proper nutrition are the only way to accomplish this.
- **It is your responsibility to be aware of how nutritious your diet is or isn't and adjust accordingly.** At times, Crohn's sufferers find the most processed foods cause the least symptoms, but it also goes without saying that these foods also provide no nutrition and are sustaining the disease and its symptoms rather than healing.

The "Normal" Standard American Diet (SAD)

With these points in mind, know that very few of us eat optimally for healing or sustaining good health. Our "normal" standard American diet is full of processed foods. Everything from animal products to vegetable oil is mass produced the cheapest way possible. All of it includes synthetic chemical compounds, hormones, pesticides, and any number of things that are toxic to our human bodies. This is not new information, but it does take a concerted effort to change the way we think and eat.

I find that changing our way of thinking is only difficult due to the culture we live in. Put another way, being "normal" and eating the SAD, including Twinkies, crackers, chips, fries, hot dogs, sodas, sugar-laden desserts, and over processed everything is only difficult until we can redefine normal. You must redefine your normal so that eating becomes a way to feed your body and provide the best possible nutrition to create healthy cells. Dairy, red meat, and grains are not bad foods. It's also true that fruits and vegetables are not always good foods. Plain and simple; foods laden with toxins or with *no* nutritional value should not be normal and <u>should be</u> avoided. This does not mean sacrificing delectable, tasty food or even the foods you enjoy. It does mean eating clean food for nutrition first and foremost.

Redefine normal so that eating becomes a way to feed your body and provide the best possible nutrition to create new healthy cells.

Four things related to diet and nutrition you *must do* to support the symptom-free lifestyle and heal your body are:

1. *Get over the idea that you eat only for pleasure.* Food should primarily be consumed to *feed your body,* not to pleasure your taste buds. Your digestive tract only knows what it can digest, use to fuel your body, and provide nutrition to the body's cells—not how good the hamburger or cookie tasted. It is also good to be aware of the fact that while your system is compromised with active disease, any filler foods that you ingest are only putting more stress on the system. The filler foods include non-nutritious, processed, and sugar-laden snacks.

2. *Stop eating any food you know is causing you present problems.* If you are running to the bathroom with each bite of ice cream, then respect yourself enough to stop eating ice cream. If your system is not healthy enough to assimilate nutrients from fresh vegetables, then stop eating those or find a different preparation for them. Until your body has less inflammation and can digest certain food again, honor the symptom and find an alternative way to get that nutrition.

Blaming or hating the disease because you can't eat foods
you think you want will not get you to a healing place.

3. *Allow yourself to eat what is best for you without self-incrimination or feeling abnormal.* It is much easier now
than it was years ago to say "I can only eat this or that" as
it is more common to have special diets. Restaurants will
accommodate most special requests without fuss, and it is
also easy to find a variety of fresh fruits, fresh vegetables,
and nutritious snacks year round at the grocery. Redefine
normal to suit you.

4. *Eat whole foods that are primarily organic.* These types of
foods are much easier on our systems than combined foods.
Whole foods are foods that exist in nature, and for the most
part we eat them as nature intended. Fruits, vegetables,
grains, nuts, and seeds and animal products such as beef,
fish, poultry, pork, and eggs are all whole foods. If it has
more than one ingredient, it will be harder to digest and may
be much less nutritious. Whole, unprocessed milk products
can also be tolerated without distress more than pasteurized
or ultra-pasteurized dairy products.

I learned a technique years ago about proper food combining that has
served me well. Combining, or as the case may be not combining,
certain foods goes a long way in my being able to eat most anything.
For example, I can easily eat baked chicken or turkey alone and I
can easily eat potatoes, *but* I cannot eat potatoes and cooked poultry
together. The symptoms they create are nausea and bloating. The
same goes for trying to combine a SAD breakfast such as oatmeal
and fruit. Grains and fruits should not be eaten together, but eaten
at different times, they can both be tolerated with fewer symptoms.

Another trick I learned was to eat smaller, more frequent portions of
food. Whether nibbling all day tricks your body into not thinking it
is eating or it is just better to have something always being digested,

I am not sure, but this reduced many of the regular symptoms of eating larger less frequent meals.

Putting It into Practice:

Step 2—Eat to Feed

There are many diet alternatives being published today: Atkins, SCD, Paleo, just to name a few. I encourage you to research and try out any and all of these to find something that will give you some immediate relief and also will work for you over time. Again, diets are specific to each of us, and there is no one answer that fits all. The step to master here about any diet, and foods in general, is to take control of what you feed your body and make it as nutritious as you can.

1. Keep a journal of everything you eat during a week's time. Next to each food, note if it is processed, whole, fresh, or filler. Also note how nutritious it is for your body. (You could use a one- to three-point system.) The idea here is to become aware of what you are actually putting in your mouth and how much nutrition it is providing for you. Over the following weeks, start replacing the least-nutritious, processed foods with whole foods. You may find it easier to do one meal at a time or just replace filler snacks with nuts, fruits, carrots, etc. Over time, with practice and determination, it will become second nature to choose good foods over bad.

2. Also note, while going through the above exercise, which foods are current triggers for your symptoms. Listen to what your body is telling you, and adjust accordingly. When the stomach ulcers are bleeding and you can't seem to eat oranges without pain, don't eat oranges.

3. Experiment with organic, whole foods, and add them to your diet as your symptoms permit. Always keep what is most nutritious to your body in the forefront of what goes in your mouth.

4. Do some studying on natural, organic nutritional supplements (do not take synthetic vitamins), food combining, and juicing. All are things that will help digestion and get more nutrition to fuel your body.

5. Grow our own garden, make your own organic probiotics like kefir or kombucha, cook more meals at home, and include your family in the processes. Adding the extra effort of love it takes to provide foods for yourself will make a difference in how you see your food.

6. Make the decision to change your diet according to the severity of current symptoms. Remember that things will be better and you will be able to eat some of those favorites you can't today.

3

Detox Your Living Environment

Environmental pollution imperils humans. This fact is well-documented.

I think we can all agree that we live in a polluted environment. Our food is produced with chemicals that are toxic to our bodies. Lotions, soaps, and laundry detergent are all harmful to our skin. People are being diagnosed with food allergies, asthma, and diabetes, all related to what we eat and breathe. We do live in a toxic environment, and the toxins in the body cause many of the diseases that medical science deals with; autoimmune diseases are no exception. One of the ways to take control of your health and reduce your symptoms is to refuse to let toxins into your life.

Simply put, your body does not know how to deal with many of the chemicals and toxins that enter it, and the digestive system is one of the hardest hit. From changing the normal bacteria flora to literally eating holes in your system, physical toxins are a major problem.

Emotional toxins are also a real threat. Stories in the evening news of our poor economy, war, and political issues create negative emotions. Our economy is tenuous at best. Money issues create stress and anxiety. All of these emotions are, over time, buried in our bodies or more pointedly in our digestive tracts.

While it would be a stretch to believe you can remove all toxins from your environment, you can consciously reduce them, which will help your healing immeasurably. Realize that as wonderful as your body is, you need to help it in any way you can, and that includes not subjecting it to chemicals it does not know how to deal with. Eliminating as many toxins as possible from your environment is one of the most challenging differences we will need to make to heal our bodies.

People can also be toxic to your lifestyle and emotions. If you have someone in your life who sabotages your attempts at a healthy diet or makes you feel less than you are, you have seen how hard that can be on you. Look inside and trust your instincts about whether you have relationships that are toxic to you. Sometimes setting boundaries is enough; sometimes ending the relationship altogether may be needed.

Putting It into Practice

Step 3—Repel Toxic Waste

This practice can be one of the most challenging. Detoxing your environment of chemicals, people, and habits will not be done overnight, and in reality is a continuous decision. With practice and clarity, it will become easier to make those everyday decisions on what you can have in your life to support your good health and what you do not want any part of.

- Go through your food cupboards and personal care items, and take note of how many chemicals are in the things you put on or in your body. You can find an organic, chemical-free option for anything you use on a daily basis. In my experience, the additional cost is not significant over the course of a lifetime, and the money you save on medications will easily cover it. There are so many excellent, organic, sustainable products that you will enjoy much more, knowing they are not poisoning your system.

- Get out and enjoy clean, fresh air, sun, and nature as often as possible. Indoor air is full of concentrated pollutants. While outdoor air can also be polluted, just being outdoors and in nature promotes good lung, blood, and digestive functions and is an instant stress reducer.

- Limit time in front of your electronic devices, including the television, computers, and video games. Radiation and electromagnetic energies wreak havoc in our bodies. Use landline phones and the speaker on your cell phone whenever possible.

- Drink clean water. And that does not always mean bottled water as there are many bottled waters that have a high numbers of toxins in them. Find a purifying system that suits your home and lifestyle.

- Medications are toxic to your body. While they may seem to be doing good things, know that they also are creating side effects. To counteract some of the side effects while taking the meds and especially after stopping them, include detoxifying foods such as ginger, green tea, aloe vera, turmeric, and lemon in your diet.

- Watch less TV. Many unrealistic beliefs about our world are attributed to fictional and even real-life negative stories in the news. Find alternative newspapers or news sites to listen to. Fill your world with good, clean messages.

- Look at your relationships with friends, family, and coworkers. How do these relationships hurt or help your healthy lifestyle? Make a decision to let in only those who support you and your healing wholeheartedly.

4

Rest Is Permissible

Give yourself permission to rest and heal.

As a society, we are very sleep deprived and put a lot of emphasis on being productive instead of taking the time needed to rest our bodies. Although scientists have just begun to identify the connections between insufficient sleep and disease, most experts have concluded that getting enough high-quality sleep is as important to health and well-being as nutrition and exercise. Study after study supports the fact that proper sleep will make us less stressed emotionally and physically, supports brain function, and gives the cells in our bodies time to reproduce efficiently. Interactions between sleep and the immune system have been well documented. Sleep deprivation increases the levels of many inflammatory issues, and inflammation and infection in turn affect the amount and patterns of sleep creating a negative circle effect.

Simply stated, sleep provides the human body with needed energy rejuvenation and frees your mind from the constant barrage of thoughts. You absolutely must give yourself permission to rest and heal. You cannot think it is selfish to take care of yourself. Those with Crohn's disease not only need the extra sleep, but it is also imperative for them to get extra rest even when they are symptom free due to their compromised immune systems.

I know there may be some of you who cannot sleep due to medications or anxiety that the disease brings about. I encourage you to keep looking for ways to give both your body and your mind rest. Something I did while taking medication that prevented me from sleeping was to take it at different times of day to accommodate the side effects.

On the flip side, I am sure some may be arguing that it seems all you do is sleep. But with that argument often I hear that you are still always fatigued and can't do the things you want or need to because you don't have the energy. This is an important point to address.

What is key in this situation is your *attitude* about rest and relaxing. If you are not giving yourself permission to sleep more than seven to eight or even ten hours per night or rest during the day with a grateful attitude, then it is not helping you as much as it could. *Giving yourself permission is putting yourself in the mind-set that healing comes first.* Soon enough, you will h be able to do more as your body heals. But when you need rest, rest and be okay with that.

This was one of my biggest challenges I had to learn and practice consistently over the years—to give myself permission to *rest* and then take the time to do so.

Let me explain further. As a young mother with Crohn's, I was still determined to be a supermom. At times the symptoms slowed me down considerably, and I would sleep for hours or I would take a couch break when needed, but inside, I was really *not okay with that.* I was still not able to let myself relax. Upon awakening, or while I was lying on the couch, I would think about how much I hated the disease, berated myself about all the things I did not get accomplished that day or think about the time I wasn't spending with my family or taking care of everyday activities. Sound familiar? I was resting but not relaxing. Instead of thinking what a good day it had been, I would go to sleep thinking about what I had failed to accomplish. I was hating the rest needed to heal instead of being grateful for it, so in the end it was causing me anxiety rather than helping my body. It wasn't until I gave myself permission to relax that it did me any good in managing my symptoms.

The key to this process is to give yourself permission to do less. Don't try to be the do-all and end-all of everything and everybody in your life. Whatever you need to let go of to find time to get the needed rest, let go of it. Give yourself permission to rest, relax, and be healthy. Trust that things will get better, friends and family will understand, symptoms will lessen, and you will be able to do the things you want. Be patient with yourself.

Putting It into Practice

Step 4—Do It with Care, and Sleep It Off

1. Make a list of *all* the things you do during a day. Include everything from showering in the morning, watching your favorite TV show, doing laundry, taking care of and playing with the kids, or helping coworkers with tasks at work. Divide the list into have-to-dos and want-to-dos. Do this without judgement but with some serious thought and honesty.

2. Identify two or more of the things you feel *you have to do* but could replace with some rest time or with extra sleep. To make this happen, you may need to think of ways to be more organized. Give tasks to others in the household, teach

the kids how to make their own snacks, implement specific times to answer e-mails at work, etc.

Many of the have-to-dos on your list may feel like obligations and zap your physical and emotional energy. These things need to be looked at closely as to why you feel this way, and they may need to be limited or eliminated. All activities create a stress and anxiety to a certain degree, but it is especially true when we set ourselves up to not let someone else down. Crohn's disease symptoms feed on stress and anxiety, so it just makes sense to limit the things you *feel or think* you have to do for others as much as possible.

It is good to note here that you also need to get rid of all unnecessary time commitments. It may take some time to extract yourself from some of those commitments, but start by giving yourself permission to do so. Then decide what can stay and what can go. Be ruthless, and know that you are doing this for you. Women are notorious for not saying *no* when we really should for a myriad of reasons. But men also need to look at the commitments that eat up their time and cause anxiety about "having to do."

3. Now take a hard look at the want-to-do list. Are these things you really feel you want to do, or do you, again, feel obligated or that you should do them? A good way to tell the difference here is by your excitement level. Typically, things you want to do will excite you, and you find the energy and enthusiasm to do them, whereas the obligations or "shoulds" will drain your energy—just like the activities that you feel you have-to-do specifically for others.

Be Aware and Limit Any Shoulds

A lesson I wish I had learned much earlier in life, was that *should* was a guaranteed symptom creator for Crohn's sufferers. Anything you put with the word "should" can be eliminated from your world *or* you need to look at the action a different way. An example of seeing a situation in a different light here might be believing you "should" help your grandmother with cleaning her house even though you are tired. Instead, look at it this way, "I am glad to spend time with my grandmother, and I feel it is a gift to help her." This switch in how you look at things will have a positive effect on your emotions by taking the negativity out of many situations. Even though you may still feel physically tired, the positive emotion created will not cause stress.

Accept that even doing the want-to-dos is not always in your best interest. Give yourself permission to stay home and rest, trusting that your family and friends want the best for you and will understand. Trust that things will get better, symptoms will lessen, and you will be able to do the things you want. Patience with yourself is part of giving that permission to sleep, rest, and heal. This loving act towards yourself will go far in your healing.

It is your loving lifestyle changes that make the real difference in improved health.

THE EMOTIONAL
STRESSES

Just like any disease, Crohn's disease can be emotionally trying, *but* unlike most diseases, I have come to realize that many of the symptoms (or lack of them) have a direct relationship *to* your emotions. Have you ever been in a situation where you have had a reaction of a sudden tightness or uneasiness in your stomach? Have you felt a sudden nausea when confronted with a situation outside of your comfort level? This is an example of how emotions are directly related to your physical body and especially the digestive tract. Of course, most people experience these types of physical reactions to emotional situations, but Crohn's sufferers tend to take emotional reactions to the next level.

A Sensitive Type

It is a common characteristic that those with digestive issues are highly sensitive people. This is neither good nor bad, just a reality to be aware of. By definition, we try hard to be people pleasers, and we take on others' problems, emotions, and hurts. We respond by trying to fix the situations and heal the hurts and worry for them, not realizing how it is affecting us. Still be caring and compassionate, but it is best for all to stay neutral to others' emotional situations. Stated another way, your worry about the other person's situation is not helpful to you and will eventually be a cause of symptoms.

Earlier I mentioned how everything in this world is made up of energy. Emotions, problems, and feelings (both your own and others') create an energy. These energies surrounding emotions are powerful and affect your body in a myriad of ways. Negative emotions, such as fear, sadness, disappointment, or anger, most often will land in your digestive tract.

Your own emotions are created by the way you react to any given situation. When you react negatively, it creates a negative emotion, which will typically settle in your gut. Traumas, fears, anger, regrets, feeling overwhelmed, or criticism are some of the most common. Awareness is the first step to remedying the cause. Awareness allows you to step back and realize that the emotion of the situation needs to be released.

There are several ways to deal with your emotions that will help to heal your Crohn's disease. In this section we will explore those steps. The first is to define your why of being healthy. Then we will discover how your attitude can control the emotions to a calmer you. The later steps discuss how to make decisions that can enable you to take control of your life, thus creating a lifestyle that minimizes negativity.

5

Your Reason Why

He who has a why to live can bear almost any how.
—Friedrich Nietzsche

We all have hopes, dreams, and bucket lists—things we want to do in our lives. We also have a picture of what we want our lives to look like. When suddenly diagnosed with a disease that may forever change that picture, the shock and sadness that invokes can completely derail a person. You can suddenly feel like you are no longer in control, no longer able to make decisions about your life. The emotional turmoil looks very much like a grieving process and justifiably so. You have been thrown off your path and find yourself on a very different road, left wondering what life can hold for you now. No happiness? Endless doctor and hospital visits? Loneliness? Pain? Anger? And guilt as to what you have done wrong? The list can go on and on.

This is where you need to take an emotionally decisive action to regain your health and do what the doctors can't. You need to believe that *you are in control* of your body and well-being. It is your decision that will make the difference. If you decide to heal your body, then you can remedy the dis-ease. Provide it with the nutrition it needs, change the way you react to life circumstances, and do anything else needed. This can be an explosive emotional issue, and you will need to stand strong and enlist the help of supporters around you, but in the end it can hold the success you are looking for. You will be able to reduce the debilitating symptoms, you will heal your body (maybe not 100 percent but noticeably), and you will remain in control of your medical situation and your life.

As you decide to take control of your health, the first thing you need to identify is **your reason** *to be healthy—your* **why**. This *reason* will become your driving force to implement the healing steps over the next several weeks, months, and years. It will become the thing that reminds you to not eat the donuts when everyone else is, the thing that holds you accountable.

One of the first realizations I had after being diagnosed with Crohn's disease was I felt blessed that if I had to have a disease, it was one I considered manageable and not fatal. Sounds selfish and harsh at first, but it also shored up my decisive control. If it could be managed, then I could manage it. I also very soon realized that I had a game-changing *reason to be healthy.* In my case, this was the ability to raise my children as normally as possible. I did not want to be dependent. I did not want to be restricted in the outdoor adventures we as a family loved to partake in. I did not want to have to tell my child, no, I didn't have the energy to participate. I wanted to interact, be able to live out that life of my dreams, be a part of their lives, and do it in a healthy way. This *reason* became my driving force to do what it took to heal my body, have energy, and live a normal life. I never looked back.

Putting It into Practice

Step 5—Why Live the Life

I have made thousands of choices in regard to my own good health over the years, and all were made with my ultimate goal in mind—my why. *Your why* will keep you on the road to healing. Each mouthful of food, each decision to rest, each choice to put yourself and your health first, each relationship you nourish or run from—each time you choose to *not* let a particular situation get to you, you make with this ultimate goal in mind. You need to identify your reason *why*.

- Spend some time soul searching and thinking about all that you are thankful for in your life.
- Make your bucket list.
- Identify the things, people, and reasons you want to be healthy.
- What are your hopes and dreams?
- Identify what drives you to be you.
- What is your game changer in the things you have identified as important to you? It needs to be something that is so important your life would have no meaning without it.
- What is the reason for the nonnegotiable contract you are willing to make with yourself to make the needed changes that will heal your body?
- Why do you want this?

Write down your why, text it to your friends and family, make a poster for the kitchen wall, and look at it every day. Going forward, whenever you feel that you cannot go on, the road is too tough, or the choice is too hard, you will want to remember this reason to be healthy—your *why*. This is a critical step in taking control of your own health. This conviction will become your driving force to go on.

Now, believe very confidently that you can have all that you have identified you want out of life. Take a moment to picture that healthy, fun-loving person enjoying life and living the dreams. It is a life that is not restricted by diet, pain, or embarrassing symptoms and that is happy, with wonderful relationships and all the success you can dream of. When you can see yourself living the life of your dreams, you begin to change your beliefs, and the positive emotions begin to heal the dis-ease. It will take time and effort, some bad days, and some setbacks but in the end you will have the life that you picture. Your why will keep you on track. I promise that it will make a difference.

6

An Attitude of Gratitude

The struggle ends when the Gratitude begins.
—Neale Donald Walsch

As I have said, Crohn's disease is very much an emotional disease. Emotions—happiness, sadness, contentment or discontent with life, stress, anxiety, depression, happiness, and appreciation are all game changers in our disease management. Internalized negative emotions cause dis-ease, resulting in symptoms and a diseased body.

Emotions stem from your reactions and create an attitude. In any given moment, about any given thing, we as humans have a reaction (usually a gut reaction) that in turn forms a belief and then an attitude about the situation. As with any disease, and especially with digestive diseases, you can worsen or improve your symptoms immeasurably depending on your attitude. A good attitude can counteract those negative emotions that would eventually land in our digestive tract.

I have found that there are several techniques to change our attitudes. Practicing patience and faith, building self-confidence, looking at others with compassion, or stepping into their shoes are some that you can develop.

But I have found that the number-one technique for getting our attitudes where they need to be to *improve* our symptoms is *gratitude*. It gets us away from blame, anger, judgement, and fear and any other negative emotion you can think of. When you can honestly be thankful for not only the good things in your life and the people who you love but also the challenges, pain, and discomfort or less-liked people, you are on the right road—the road to health.

It took me several years into my diagnosis before I could really be grateful for my disease and my symptoms and to understand how to use that gratitude to help myself. As I became more and more aware of what was causing my symptoms and realized that it was my body's way of telling me something, I was able to react more and more quickly to controlling the symptom. As time went on, this became a telling circle and one of the most important aspects of my good health. Bad attitudes led to stress and anger that would affect my gut, which led to symptoms of pain and diarrhea. The symptoms made me realize something was wrong that I needed to correct. Being grateful for the symptoms gave me the ability to realize it was my negative attitude that needed to change. This gave me reason to work on whatever was troubling me, which put me back into good health.

Putting It into Practice

Step 6—It's All Attitude

1. The first thing to bless is conventional medicine. Actually say *out loud* thank you for medicines, doctors, and procedures for providing you with some relief. Realize that you need these things at this moment in your life. You will not always need them, but they are here for you now, so say thank you!

2. Make a list of no less than twenty-five things you are grateful for right now in your life—big things, small things, and those you wouldn't think to bless. It would serve you best to do this at least weekly going forward. A daily gratitude moment is even more helpful.

   My gratitude list would include: family, a warm home, ability to make money, technology to interact with others easily, the ability to eat horseradish (I love horseradish), aloe vera, mountain blue skies, snow, warm beaches, flannel sheets, holding grandbabies … you get the idea.

3. Now, discover what things you are grateful for about your disease. This is a two-part process. First, I want you to list the symptoms you are experiencing currently and then list why you are grateful for that symptom. For example, your list may look something like this:

   • Diarrhea … thank you gut for alerting me to the fact that I have let this part of my body reach such an inflamed state that it cannot function correctly and will cause me to be malnourished and dehydrated. *Or* thank you, gut, for alerting me to the fact that I cannot digest this food right now and it does me *no* good to put it in my mouth.

   • Aching joints and legs … thank you, nerves, for alerting me that even though I may not be having any gut symptoms, my body is experiencing some inflammation that it is fighting.

   • Intestinal blockage … thank you, gut, for alerting me to the fact that I may not be eating enough fiber to pass foods easily. (Or whatever the solutions need to be.)

It may be hard at first to bless your disease and the symptoms, but with practice you will be able to see that your body is just trying to help you be conscious of its problems. You need to respond with gratitude and then the willingness to do what it takes to fix the problem. Bless your body and say thank you for the messages it is sending you. Do this every day for the rest of your life.

There is one more point I want to make on attitude and emotions. I found that the best way to counteract negative emotions that were spiraling me down a wrong road was to take *positive* action. As my deliberate positive actions went up, the negative emotions went down. When I was insecure, lonely, frustrated, judgmental, hateful, sad, or fearful, I would push myself to take action to counteract the emotion. Sadness left me when I hugged my kids. Lonesomeness went away when I talked to a friend. Fear subsided with a trip to the library or now googling ways to address the problem I was fearful of. Self-development courses created security and confidence. The actions kept the negative emotions from settling in my gut and prevented them from causing symptoms. Over time this became a learned response, and I was able to quickly see what action I needed to take.

7

Help Yourself— the Decision to Heal

Make the decision to accept responsibility and take control of your own health.

Helping yourself is not just about getting to the doctor consistently or asking the right questions. Nor is it just about making sure you rest when needed or eat the most nutritious foods. These everyday needs are important, but what I am talking about is the bigger picture. It is the *decision* that you are in control and you will help yourself.

This decision comes with responsibility. You must first acknowledge and come to terms with yourself that there are aspects of your lifestyle that have gotten you to this place of disease. Most of these aspects come from no conscious fault of your own. Your personality type is a factor. The foods you eat, the lifestyle you lead, or the unknowingness of living in a toxic environment can all contribute. Just not knowing there is a different way to heal other than conventional medicine is a big factor. You may not have been aware of all these issues until now.

The responsibility now becomes yours to turn your disease, symptoms, and healing around. If you are really honest with yourself, it is my guess that this awareness is only a confirmation of something you already knew or had inklings of. It came as no big surprise to me that when I changed my lifestyle and took care of myself, with my healing as the objective, it changed my symptoms. You no doubt also know there are things you are doing today that are not in your best interest where your disease is concerned, and these things are causing your symptoms.

The great part is that it is never too late to change your life. No matter where you are today … making the decision and taking the responsibility to take care of *you* is a *huge* step to healing. It may not be easy, but make the decision to help yourself. Take back your life and your body, and most importantly, change the habits that got you to the dis-eased place you are in. I made the commitment to help myself, and you can too. I trusted in myself and believed in myself first and foremost, and I did not rely just on the doctors or medications to heal my disease.

The reality check I had when I made this decision was that it was the food I was eating. It was the physical stress I was putting myself through. It was the emotional issues of unhappiness and feeling I was lacking something in my life. It was the fears of inadequacy I was swallowing. It was the feeling I had no control and was fated to be sick. It was wanting to continually please others and failing. I literally had *caused* my symptoms to flourish, and my digestive tract had weakened. I realized I needed to change my habits and the way I dealt with my emotions. It was hard to look at myself and take that responsibility, but it is a crucial step.

The decision to take responsibility and then care for yourself can be an uncomfortable one—especially for those who have been diagnosed with a disease. It is easy to get caught up in, "Why me?"

and "What did I do to deserve this?" or "It is just bad luck, and I have to deal with it." This is a line of questioning that, while essential for our psyche to ask initially, does more harm than good when we dwell on it. To dwell there makes us the victim and keeps those negative emotions fed. It takes away our power to thrive and do something about helping ourselves heal.

We are raised to depend on others for our well-being, and we live in a culture that is continually trying to convince us to think that someone else knows best. From the time we were infants, we have been taught to take others' direction and advice before our own intuition and knowing. Seldom do we hear that our decisions and ideas are good, are complimented on what we do know, or are allowed the freedom to listen to our inner knowing. Instead, we have been conditioned into always relying on others and to believe someone else knows best.

- ✓ Conventional medicine has us going to the doctor with the first sign of illness—even a common cold.
- ✓ You need only to turn on the TV to see how the latest product will make you better, faster, prettier, stronger, etc.
- ✓ Do this, do that, and you will be a better this and that … the examples are endless.

What I want to impress on you, is that only you—with the proper information and discernment—know what is best for you. Many of us will ignore that small voice that warns us that something isn't good for us and follow blindly. We all have an intelligence and an intuition that serves us well, and it is wise to develop the art of listening to it. You have the power to change your habits, heal your body, and become better in the process just by listening to that inner voice.

Making the decision to take control of your health is a huge leap of faith. Your health is your business, but the insecurity in that can be a constant companion. You need to stay strong and decide that you will do whatever it takes to help yourself be healthy and live the life you want. It is your body, your life, and your disease to deal with. No one knows better what is best for you than you. When you can accept responsibility and decide to take care of yourself, you are on the path to health.

Trust yourself to take care of you.

Putting It into Practice

Step 7—Trust You to Help You

1. Make a conscious, *out loud* decision that you are going to take care of you by making your body well and doing what it takes to stay that way. *Decide today* that while you may take advice from doctors, family, and other IBD patients, you will *only do what is right for you*. Accept that responsibility for *you*.

2. Look at your current prescribed routine—medications, diets, follow-up visits, tests, etc.—and decide what *is* working and what *is not* working for you. Are there possible alternatives you need to look at?

   One of the things I took control of in my own health regimen was to reduce the number of colonoscopies from what the GI (who I loved, by the way) wanted me to take as routine follow-ups. Just the idea of the test would remind me of my disease. If I wasn't experiencing any symptoms and was feeling fine, the fear of the test and the prep was enough to send me into a major flare. I made the decision to only deal with the GI doctor if I was having problems that I felt would spiral downward. Otherwise, I depended on myself to right what needed to change and put myself back on a healthy path. This served me well, not self-diagnosing but by being aware of my reactions, attitude, and lifestyle that caused my symptoms.

3. Identify some of the main complaints you have about your disease and how you might become more educated to help yourself reduce or heal those issues. Understand the idea of dis-ease of your body, take nutrition classes, read up on alternative diets, practice meditation, or take a self-development course. Go on a mission to learn whatever you feel unsure of and gain the working knowledge you need to responsibly take care of you.

8

Look at Your Life

The lifestyle you have led or are leading
has gotten you to this place of dis-ease.

To make a healthy lifestyle change, you need to know where you are right now and what things have contributed to your symptoms and disease. You will need to take stock of what is causing more stress, less stress, more happiness, or more sadness and disappointment. When you can see your life very clearly, you can pinpoint the changes that need to be made.

Ulcers in your stomach or lower intestines don't just happen, and it is a lifestyle issue, reaction, or attitude that has caused your body to eat itself up. Emotions that are swallowed or fears that are not voiced are some of the things we don't even realize we are doing to ourselves. Overwork to provide for our families or a constant drive without seeing success can wreak havoc physically.

Over time, when my symptoms were at their worst, I could always, without fail, pinpoint the things I was doing or the emotions I was feeling that were the cause of my gut symptoms. Sometimes it was diet, and at times it was major events such as a daughter leaving for college or a pet dying. And while many symptoms can come on immediately (e.g., milk products causing diarrhea), there are many more that are a slow build. Oftentimes it was the smaller things that I overlooked and just dealt with that built up into problems—things like behaviors of family members, or choices that I made that didn't set well with me. My reactions to the world around me also played a contributing factor, and I learned to not place myself in the position to be subjected to the constant barrage of negativity when needed.

People diagnosed with Crohn's disease typically have two personality traits that can be our undoing. First, as I talked about before, we are without a doubt highly sensitive people. Because we are so tuned into others, we feel their pain and are sensitive to the world around us. Internalizing others' emotions and letting them sit in our bodies can be a huge cause of our symptoms and are things to be aware of. Our own emotions need to be acknowledged also.

Second, it is common to have what is called a type A personality. Typically, we put ourselves under much stress and anxiety because we feel we must contribute, live up to others' expectations or "get it done" at all costs, which results in constant anxiety.

People with this personality will often lessen or ignore the things that make them smile. They feel the lighter emotions can waste their time or are never enough. Interestingly enough, it is also a trait in a type A personality that they have no patience in others. This judgmental impatience contradicts the sensitivity and increases the negative emotions swallowed. If you see yourself in either, or both, of the highly sensitive or the Type A get-it-done at all cost personalities, it is a good awareness. While neither of these personality traits is bad, they will contribute to your disease symptoms and an internalizing of emotions if you are not careful.

Awareness and acknowledgment are the first steps to being able to know where you need to change. Take a look at your life—the things you spend your time doing, how you feel, and why you feel that way. Be brutally honest and nonjudgmental in your assessments of time and feelings. This is the only way to get to the underlying emotions (positive and negative) that are either helping to improve your symptoms or are causing your issues.

Putting it into Practice

Step 8—Take off the Rose-Colored Glasses

Look at the life you are leading, and be brutally honest as to where your emotions are. Some things to ask yourself are:

- Are there things that need saying to your spouse, your mom, or your boss to clear the air?
- Are you disappointed with the way things have turned out in your career?
- Have you settled for something less than you desire and deserve?
- Are you living in a home that suits you, or are the apartment neighbors driving you nuts?
- Do the important people in your life support or demean you?
- Do you wish you could work full time rather than be a stay-at-home mom?
- Do you want to be a stay-at-home dad?
- What issues do you tend to ignore that you should stand your ground in?
- Is there a different schedule for work, family, and fun times that would better suit you?
- Is money an issue? Do you have the freedom to earn, spend, and save? Do you want that freedom or be financially supported?
- Do you find yourself constantly apologizing to others?

- Are you successful but unfulfilled in your career?
- Do you get the rest you feel you need?
- Do you overschedule yourself? Do you feel a need to contribute to the point of exhaustion?
- Are your children overscheduled?
- Do you eat foods you shouldn't because it is easier?
- Do you feel you neglect your children?
- Is your spiritual faith in a higher power solid? Missing? Nurtured?
- Do you feel insecure in you?
- Do you feel guilty that you do not know how to cook? Keep house? Make more money?
- Do you trust your doctor but feel there is more he should be doing?

As you go through this exercise and look at your life, be honest as to where your emotions are sitting for each issue you identify. You may find that it is uncomfortable and difficult. Just awareness of the issues can release some of the internalized emotions, and you may find yourself angry, hurt, frustrated, or feeling any other negative emotion coursing through you. You may start to experience pain or other symptoms.

If this becomes the case, remember to stop and do the following:

1. Bless the symptom, and realize the strength in that awareness.
2. Realize that you cannot change what you are not aware of.
3. See that your emotions are a direct result of your reaction to the situation.

You will heal your body by changing your reactions and attitude. Right now you need to know where you are and what you are feeling. Remember to also practice the gratitude we talked of earlier while going through this exercise. Saying thank you for the clarity a situation brings you will move your attitude to one of control and positive action to do something about it.

It is important to note the circumstances in your life that are going right also. Recognize, take stock, and brainstorm all the good things, accomplishments, loving friends, and family you have too. Notice how you feel when you think about these things. Note your attitude, emotions, and physical symptoms. If you are smiling, your digestive tract is too.

9

Turn 180 degrees

What puts a smile on your face? You need a lot of that.
What makes you spitting mad? You need a lot less or
none of that.

Now that you have taken a hard look at your life, it is time to do
something about it; take action and make changes. This next step
down our path of self-healing is to identify where we need to turn
180 degrees. Now is the time to decide how you want to change the
areas of our life you don't like (i.e., the ones that literally make you
sick). You also need to commit do more of the things that make you
smile.

Your life is for you to create. If, up to now, you have felt that your
life has been decided for you by fate, think again. If you believe that
the best anyone can do is go down the road they have been put on,
then you need to know you are wrong. You are the creator of your
life, and unless you like that road you feel you have been put on, the
time to change is now. No one makes the choices but you. What you
choose to spend your time doing, and how you react to the life you
have created is of utmost importance. Are you going to settle for or
justify the road you are on *or* see it for what it really is (a symptom
maker) and change course *now*? There is so much to learn, to enjoy,

to be pleased with. There are so many good people to support you and so many things to have fun doing. Choose those things that make you smile. Reach for and complete that bucket list.

> *Twenty seconds of insane courage. Just literally twenty seconds of just embarrassing bravery, and I promise you something great will come of it.*

This is a quote from the popular movie *We Bought a Zoo*. I find it very relevant here because very often change takes so much courage that we just don't do it. We instead revert to blaming others or the universe and try to make the best of bad situations. This creates emotional distress for ourselves and what does that do? It is a wicked merry-go-round that is not merry at all.

I want you to know that this is often the hardest step to accomplish. Many times we know situations are wrong in our lives and recognize that they are contributing to our dis-ease but would rather not rock the boat or find the courage to change them. It is hard to change when it affects others around you. It is hard to turn around and follow a new path, scary to leave the known and comfortable. But I am here to tell you that everything you have identified that is creating negativity in your life will be better gone. Finding a new job, packing up the house for a move, confronting relatives, or distributing new chores to family members is hard work, and it will weaken your resolve. It takes courage. And it is here that you need to remember these things:

1. Think of your *why*—your reason to be healthy
2. Be grateful for the clarity these situations have given you
3. Detoxing your life is a must to get an upper hand on healing
4. Situations that you are unhappy with are causing negative emotions, which is causing your disease.
5. Courage and security come with positive action.

Putting It into Practice

Step 9—Flip It

1. Use the things you identified earlier when taking a hard look at your life. For every item identified that you may not be pleased with and that creates a negative emotion, write a corresponding note as to what you will do to turn that 180 degrees. Some things may be quick and easy, like finding a new apartment away from noisy neighbors, or they may take some time, such as going back to school to have that career you want. Sometimes it does not take a physical change at all but a change in your emotional reaction to a situation. Start slow or hit sixty in sixty seconds, but start today. Your quality of life—your symptom-free life—depends on it.

2. For each item identified as something that makes you happy, decide how to work it into your life as often as possible. If it is a relationship, then nurture it. If it is training for a marathon, then run as much as you are able. Celebrating the good things over and over allows you to easily create the attitudes of gratefulness and happiness that will heal you.

By the way … taking the step to learn more about your disease and the ways to become symptom free and take control of your health is an amazing step you can be proud of right now.

10

Setting Boundaries

Setting boundaries for yourself is one of the most loving things you can do.

The time will come when you will begin to feel better, your symptoms will be less severe or nonexistent, and you will be in what the doctors refer to as a remission. You will be able to refer to this time as *feeling amazingly good*! But the ultimate goal in your symptom-free lifestyle is not to get you to a remission but to make it sustainable over the rest of your life. What does it take to keep the disease at bay forever?

Of course, implementing lifestyle changes to reduce stress on your body and doing things that make you happy will keep you on course, but often we fall back into old patterns when we are feeling better, and then a familiar cycle reemerges. Suddenly your symptoms have returned, and even though maybe not as bad as before, you get that sinking feeling of dis-ease again.

How many times have you felt better for months, only to decide that you can take on those extra three classes at college and then fall victim to the anxiety of getting all A's? Or maybe you have taken a new job and with the new time constraints you find yourself not eating anything but fast food? Or a common thing when you have been symptom free for an extended length of time is to have your friends, family and/or spouse start making demands on you that they didn't before. They "forget" you have a disease and may start expecting more of your time and energy. This is where setting boundaries comes in.

The time to set boundaries and create your sustainable, healthy lifestyle is now when you are thinking about it and feeling not quite as healthy as you would like. While your symptoms are lessened but still bothering you is a perfect time to decide how to make them not come back. You do not want to fall into the cycle of "You feel better, forget everything you have been doing to help yourself, and then feel worse again."

If you are currently struggling with acute symptoms and just getting past, "How do I need to eat differently?" do not worry, come back to this step later or start thinking ahead. Remember, this is about your whole life, and you have plenty of time to master these steps. Start to think about sustainability now so you can have a roadmap later. This not just a two weeks and be done with it process. This is a lifetime commitment to take control of your own health.

So what do I mean by boundaries? These are the spectrum of practices that you will keep yourself within to stay healthy. On one end, the boundaries you set will help you to say *no* to things that you *may* think you feel well enough to do. On the opposite end of the spectrum are your lifestyle enhancers. The enhancers are the things you do to specifically take care of you.

Putting It into Practice

Step 10—the Lines to Not Cross

Make your own list as to what lines you will not cross going forward to maintain your health and healing. This is a powerful exercise, and it will give you confidence, determination, and ground to stand on when the issue needs to be faced, as it will at some point. All of the realizations, knowledge, and choices you make to keep yourself healthy come down to the boundaries you set and the ability to stand your ground.

Examples of some boundaries you may set are:

- limiting or never eating the specific foods that are known triggers for you.
- not volunteering for more than one organization at a time to concentrate your efforts and not create a situation where you are overwhelmed
- put yourself before others when it comes to your energy allowance.
- not being a doormat that makes you feel unappreciated
- not letting others coerce you into eating or doing something not in your best interest just to save face

Now think about some specific actions you can do to take care of *you*. Give yourself permission and then decide on a few lifestyle enhancers that you feel comfortable with today, and take the steps to implement those. These can change, expand, or be irrelevant at different times during your life, so treat this as a continual working list.

Examples of lifestyle enhancers are the following:

- This book and any others like it. New knowledge is a lifetime enhancer. Each time you learn something new, you will be at a different place in your health and lifestyle. You will feel different physically. You will have had some successes and some life-changing aha's. Make the promise to yourself to never stop learning.

- A good medical massage therapist. Massage is not just about relaxing muscles—even though this is a *great* way to relieve tension, stress, and anxiety. A good therapist will be able to move energy around in the body and release many of the physical and emotional traumas and toxins that collect in your gut. Set up a recurring appointment that you do not have to think about and are able to make a habit.
- A positive support system. Engage in groups or with people that support a positive lifestyle. The naysayers and worry warts will always be there, but you need people around you who are in tune with you—who sing your song or sing the song you want to hear. Remember, positive thoughts and emotions are amazing medicines and will keep you healthy. A note of caution: even though it may seem noble to join a Crohn's disease support group, pay close attention that it does not become a negative situation. You want to get away from thinking about your disease all the time, and often groups like this tend to wallow in their misery. Instead join a group that supports your new lifestyle.
- Studying current, good, unbiased medical information. Never stop learning about your disease, but do not dwell on it either. Concise information that informs and can be used as the situation warrants is good to have.
- Self-development courses that you can relate to. We are all on a different path and in a different place in our self-development. There are so many good healers and self-development books that can give you just the insight you need in your world and that will speak to where you are. The bottom line is to create a fulfilling, happy life. Develop a better you.
- A good life coach to help you through the emotional traumas and lifestyle changes you need help with. This disease will leave scars not only in your intestines but in your emotional health as well, and it may support your efforts to have a third party that supports you.

11

Cravings, Impulses, and Addictions

It is powerful medicine to do for yourself what makes you healthy.

Cravings, impulses, and addictive behaviors are things you want to be aware of in yourself and take control of. I won't go deep into the psychology of these behaviors but just touch the surface as it contributes to our needed lifestyle changes. These three behaviors stem from a sense of lack. When you feel you lack something, it becomes an anxiety in your system. Anxiety is one of those negative emotions that is a trigger of Crohn's symptoms.

Addictions such as drugs, smoking, drinking, and overeating the wrong foods are even more pronounced and physically unhealthy due to the struggle your body goes through on a daily basis. These are things to either stop completely or do in moderation if possible. I trust, since this is true of most people, that at some point in your life you have either already accomplished giving up an addiction or are well aware you need to stop. If you have beat an addiction, it is a success you should celebrate! Whether you did it because you had to (hard to smoke in the hospital or overeat when food makes you ill) or it was a choice you made and succeeded in, realize that you did this to *take care of you.* You already know how to do it and know that it can be accomplished, so there is no need to carry any addictions forward. Decide to take the steps needed to stop any bad habits.

Cravings typically come from an emotional response to a feeling of deprivation. Cravings can be physical and come from a nutritional lack in your system or from an emotional need, so notice what you are craving and why. If it serves you positively, then give into the need but in moderation. I have learned that in moderation I can tolerate many things I crave that can cause symptoms if overdone. This results in not having to deprive myself completely of something I enjoy.

One of the things I felt very deprived of at times as a young mother and began to crave was traveling. I began to feel very resentful and at times hated being home, taking those feelings out on the family or swallowing the guilt associated with that. When I pushed the point and we did take a trip, of course with our family in tow, I would inevitably return home exhausted and weak. I found that I could curb the need (craving) to get away by taking short day trips with my husband or girlfriends and still return home able to care for my family. This was such a positive change in so many ways that I overcame the craving by replacing it with something even better.

Impulses tend to originate from being out of control, unfocused, or stressed out. It is a desire that you think, at the time, will make you feel better—either emotionally or physically. Typically, on impulse you reach for something unhealthy because it satisfies that emotional need to replace the lack of control. We all tend to give in to impulses from time to time, but they will often make you feel bad emotionally if you are not careful. Of course, we do not want to go there as the downward spiral will throw you off the path of the symptom-free lifestyle you are working so hard at. Impulses can be managed by training yourself to think of something else or indulge yourself with something healthy.

When I felt I was overwhelmed, my impulse was to buy a large mocha latte. It would cause immediate reaction in my healthy stomach and always made me feel mad at myself to have eaten something I knew would hurt me. I learned to limit the impulse first by keeping ahead of my schedule and second by replacing the coffee with a piece of a dark chocolate bar. It wasn't the mocha latte I needed so much as the comfort of doing something for myself and indulging. The chocolate provided a healthier alternative to the dairy-filled coffee and was a way of taking care of and indulging me.

Addictions, cravings, and impulses can be overcome with a little practice. As your mind gets stronger, your resolve to feel good grows, and your determination becomes the norm in your healthy lifestyle, you will be able to control any impulses and cravings that can cause symptoms. The goal here is to create a lifestyle free from all the debilitating Crohn's symptoms. Do not sabotage your efforts in other areas by doing things you know are harmful to your body. Take control of your wants, desires, cravings, impulses, and addictive behaviors. Be in control of your emotions and your actions, and know how they will affect your gut. Do not use the disease or the bad behavior to justify either one or the other. Not only will you feel empowered and happy with yourself, but you will also be healthier for it.

Putting It into Practice

Step 11—Take Control

Make a list of behaviors that may be causing some of your symptoms or you know are triggers but you do anyway. Ask yourself why you are doing these things. Are there healthier choices you can make to help yourself not to feel deprived?

Your awareness will help you remember that the behavior causes the pain, and it will get easier and easier to not do. Start small and pick one thing that you can make a decision on to stop. Stick to it until you feel in control, and then choose another to work on if need be.

12

Get Outside of Yourself— Law of Attraction

Whatever you're thinking about is literally like planning a future event. When you're worrying, you are planning. When you're appreciating you are planning ... What are you planning?
—*Abraham Excerpted from: Silver Spring, MD on April 19, 1997*

While you may not buy into the universal laws (a.k.a., "the Secret" or any of the other like teachings) wholeheartedly, I am here to tell you that the universal law of attraction is very real, especially in the case of a chronic disease. Simply stated the law of attraction says, "Like attracts like" or what you think about you get. How this is important to you is that when you are only focused on your disease and its symptoms, it is what you will attract back—more disease and symptoms. Worrying constantly about being ill or needing a bathroom will make those worries come true.

If you can get outside of yourself, your symptoms, your distressing life, and your negative emotions and concentrate on happiness, caring, pain-free hours, enjoying others, etc., you will feel exponentially better. Again, what you concentrate on will come back to you.

It is important to your well-being to surround yourself with positive people, activities you enjoy, and a happy lifestyle so that you have something other to think about than your diseased digestive tract. When you are in a good mood and thinking good thoughts, you feel healthier, and that is what will come back to you—feeling healthier. Adversely, if you are laying at home watching TV, bemoaning the fact that you have a diseased gut, are tired, and have no friends who understand, you will feel all of that ill health and more.

One of the easiest ways I have found to create a feeling of well-being is to give it to others. Being of service to others by volunteering, being part of a cause, or joining an organization will not only serve the world but will give you a sense of purpose outside of yourself. It will give you something other to focus on besides your symptoms, and it will most likely become one of your reasons to be healthy. Feed your passions by serving in that capacity.

With this being said, remember to perform service with passion and a happiness of wanting to give. Do not do it from the "should" place or out of obligation. Also, do not go overboard to the point of exhaustion and feeling overwhelmed. While it is not always easy to participate if you are not feeling well, pick something that you can enjoy immensely with little or a variable time commitment. By giving to others, you give to yourself on your road to a sustainable, healthy lifestyle. Service to others became an important commitment on my want-to-do list. I created the time and did what I needed to do to have the energy to be involved.

Putting It into Practice

Step 12—Like Attracts Like

1. Pay attention to your thoughts. Our lives are created by our thoughts, and what we are thinking about comes back to us without fail. Worry and other negativity will create more problems and continue the cycle of dis-ease in your body. In choosing to be healthy and live that happy, healthy life, think those thoughts as often as possible.

2. What are some organizations or causes you can become passionate about being involved in? Reach out to people you can help and support and who provide you with good positive interaction. Doing for others is doing for you. Make it an outpouring of loving support so that it becomes one of your reasons to be healthy. Find enjoyment and satisfaction in giving to others so that the sense of well-being you give will come back to you. Get outside of yourself.

I recently heard a story of a successful businessman, author, and motivational speaker who when he was eighteen made the decision to give one-quarter of his time to volunteering in the community. What an outpouring of love and getting outside of himself that was over his lifetime. Think about how many hours less you would be thinking about or feeling your disease if your mind was engaged in serving others and creating joy around you. Give the gift of service, love, and happiness to others so it can come back to you.

13

Reevaluate

Our lives change, it seems at times, on a moment's notice. Rarely do things go along smoothly for very long. On the flip side, we tend to get into habits that we become either hesitant to change or we just don't think about anymore. Managing your disease is a lifelong process, and sustainable healing will take an everyday effort. The steps we have taken thus far are healing and management tools to address the causes of the dis-ease in your body. It will be to your advantage to create a routine evaluation, to take stock and reassess your lifestyle choices. Situations and circumstances are in continual movement, making changes in your life. What may have worked for you last year or even last month may not be working for you today.

It is an essential step to evaluate what is working and what is not. Just like medications that suddenly seem to stop having any affect, you may find that lifestyle choices stop working too. You may find that after a fulfilling career, you may want to try owning your own business, only to find that you are happier working for a nonprofit. Or maybe the easygoing people you enjoyed volunteering with are now expecting more and you feel overbooked and overstressed. Or the juicing regimen you were on is suddenly creating distress. The idea here is to not be afraid of changing over again and give yourself permission to do that without any recrimination.

I remember at one point in my life, I took a part-time position to pay off some debt. I worked there for only six weeks due to a personality clash with the owner. Even though it allowed me a good extra income and the schedule was ideal, the stress of me trying to get along with an unorganized person and compromising my integrity was not worth the money or the stress on my body. Amidst having to explain my decision to the company and then to friends who thought I was being irresponsible, I stuck to my principles of taking care of me first. By reevaluating my decision quickly, I could foresee that this position would eventually cause me Crohn's symptoms and health issues. I found another position that was much more suited to me.

Reassess and reevaluate the whole of your life often, taking new actions and directions when needed to sustain healing and wellness. It is always the right time to make some changes. The goal is to create a lifestyle of taking care of yourself, and whatever that requires today is what is right.

Putting It into Practice

Step 13—Stop, Rewind, Replay

Set aside an hour each month to reevaluate your life. Go through these steps, and touch on each of them to reassess where you are at today.

- Have you been lazy or successful about keeping most of the toxins out of your life?
- Are you eating more whole foods than processed?
- Have you been getting the rest you need?
- How you are spending your time?

- Is there just one thing you could change to make things better?
- Are the boundaries you set still relevant?
- Is there a life enhancer you recently heard about you feel you need to start?
- Are you celebrating your successes?
- Is there something you need to say no to when asked again?
- Is there something you need to say yes to?

Carve out at least fifteen minutes each day to just be with your thoughts. This can be while meditating or while you drive home, but be conscious of you and how your life is feeling. Many times just this process alone will give valuable insight.

- What are you grateful for, and what is going right?
- How did you react to people today?
- How do you feel physically? Better or worse than last week?
- How do you feel mentally?
- Are you feeling fulfilled from activities and successes today or frustrated and angry?
- Are you happy or just hanging on by your fingertips?

Knowing where you are today to begin this journey of healing and then reassessing your progress is important in the long-term sustainable lifestyle we are creating. It is human nature to take the easy road and to get stuck in outdated habits. Not taking the time to reevaluate the things you are doing after implementing these healing steps initially will not sustain the good health you are seeking throughout your life. It is especially important to stop and rewind if you are beginning to have returning symptoms.

In the End—Be Happy

Be your best self. Take care of you first. Love those around you. Be happy.

My goal for you is to heal your body and live a healthy life with Crohn's disease, symptom free and happy. Everyone on the planet has something that is amiss with their health; most just don't know it. As Crohn's patients we have the blessing of knowing exactly what hurts, and with a little awareness, we know what causes it. We also can make lifestyle and healing choices to reverse the dis-ease and ill-health. Sometimes the changes require much effort and hard choices, but with time you can begin to see the whole of the journey as a way to live your life.

The final step in your symptom-free lifestyle is to be happy. I am telling you to do what it takes to make yourself happy. Let go of any shoulds, let go of the outdated beliefs, let go of all the negative emotions that are both caused by and cause of this disease. This is not to say be mean to others for your sake or at all costs, but do have an awareness of your health first.

It may come as a real surprise to know that when you are happy, the world around you becomes happy. You attract happy people, and you make people happy. It is a simple concept, but so many miss it. Many of us are programmed to believe that we need to work to make others happy. Just the opposite is true. If you make yourself happy first with enough rest, compassion, love, gratitude, good foods, and a clean body, then others around you will be happy too, as they receive all of the same.

Many feel their Crohn's symptoms are justified, that this is their cross to bear, or that as humans we need to struggle, and you have been given this particular struggle. This is so not the case, and you need to let go of that idea first and foremost if you are going to heal. Crohn's disease and its symptoms can be managed and overcome, and through recognizing what the causes are, you can heal your body. Remember, we are the creators of our lives, and in so being, can create a healthy lifestyle that sustains a healthy body.

Has my life always been happy? Will yours always be happy if you follow this path? No, of course not, but I have found that when adverse things do come around, it is best to see what the message is and react accordingly. Being content and happy or upset and feeling lousy is all about attitude. I could be miserable over a circumstance for years or decide to quickly shake it off by replacing negative emotions with positive action and by moving in a new direction. After becoming aware, there is always the choice to either let those negative emotions and energies stay in your digestive tract or choose to let them go.

I believe we all have a responsibility to ourselves to allow ourselves to be happy. Sometimes it takes work, and sometimes it takes a little faith in ourselves or determination to move forward. Sometimes we have to buck the trend and hang out on a limb alone, but in the end it is worth the decisions you make. In so doing you become your best self.

Most times the decisions I made to make myself happy included what was best for my family and others around me. You will not be happy if you are acting from a selfish attitude or unloving place. Be strong, but be gentle and loving in everything you do.

Part of being happy is to be able to accept and love yourself for who and what you are right now. If you are not all you want to be, then do what you need to grow, but do not have anything but love for yourself at all times. We are all unique, and your lifestyle and life will never look exactly like another's. You are perfect just the way you are. Smile at that face in the mirror.

Putting It into Practice

In the End—Be Happy

Put all the steps together to *be happy, heal your body, and live symptom free.*

*Face your reality. Live by a common denominator of love. Take medications with a grain of salt. Eat to feed. Repel all types of toxic waste from your life. Do it with care and sleep it off as needed. Know **why** you want to live your desired life. Put your trust in you to help you. Stop looking through rose-colored glasses. Flip 180 degrees. No crossing the lines, and stay within your boundaries. Take control of the things that may be controlling you. Remember, like attracts like, and think only about what you really want. Stop, rewind, and replay often. Live your life to the fullest, but do so knowingly and with intention.*

I have had no formal medical training but have spent years teaching myself on a myriad of self-help issues, including Crohn's disease and its symptoms and causes. I am an accountant by trade who has turned writer and life coach, a visionary who sees the reality in believing in the power of our thoughts and emotions to create our lives and heal our bodies. I have a strong determination and a passion for showing others an alternative way to heal their bodies using awareness, natural alternatives, and nutrition, and staying away from dependency on conventional medical treatments. As I am no different from each of you who is trying to life our best life, I believe I can speak to your fears and uncertainties about this disease. I continue to live through the everyday struggles and the proof of my success is being overall symptom free and healthy after 25 plus years. These aspects of managing your life I have presented in this book developed out of need and necessity and a want for something better than I was being offered. If you can see yourself just where I was, I encourage you to gain strength and encouragement in these words from someone who understands. I want you to live your best life and do it symptom free.

For more information and to follow the Blog go to
www.livehealthywithcrohns.com